Fighting cancer: a practical guide to the symptoms, causes and treatments of cancerous diseases

Leo Raphael Pineda

Fighting cancer: a practical guide to the symptoms, causes and treatments of cancerous diseases

SUMMARY

Fighting cancer: a practical guide to the symptoms, causes and treatments of cancerous diseases

Introduction

Fighting cancer: a practical guide to the symptoms, causes and treatments of cancerous diseases

Cancer is one of the deadliest and most widespread diseases worldwide, affecting millions of people every year. The exact causes of cancer are complex and often difficult to identify, but many factors can contribute to its development, such as age, lifestyle, genetics, environment, etc.

Cancer can manifest in many ways, with different symptoms depending on the type of cancer. Some cancers are detected very early through screening programs, but others are not discovered until symptoms are more advanced.

Cancer treatment depends on the type and stage of the disease, as well as the patient's personal preferences. Treatment options may include surgery, radiation therapy, chemotherapy, immunotherapy, etc. The side effects of treatment can be very difficult for patients to manage, and the healing process can be long and difficult.

Despite advances in cancer treatment and prevention, much more needs to be done to fight this devastating disease. Healthcare professionals, researchers, patients and survivors are all working together to improve treatments and find a way to cure cancer permanently.

In this book, we will explore the different facets of

cancer disease, providing information on symptoms, causes, treatments and prevention strategies. We will also share stories of people who have been affected by cancer, to give readers a better understanding of what it is like to live with this disease.

We'll start with a detailed introduction to what cancer is, how it forms, the different types of cancer, and the most common risk factors. We will then look at the screening methods available for the different types of cancer, as well as the advantages and limitations of each method.

We'll also explore the process of diagnosing cancer, including common signs and symptoms, the most common diagnostic tests, and stages of diagnosis. We will also provide information on the different cancer treatment options, including surgery, radiation therapy, chemotherapy, and immunotherapy, as well as the side effects associated with each treatment.

We will also cover the management of common symptoms in cancer patients , such as pain, fatigue, weight loss, etc. We will provide practical advice to help patients manage these symptoms, so they can live the most comfortable life possible during their treatment.

Finally, we'll discuss life after treatment, including the long-term effects of cancer and its treatments, as well as monitoring and preventing recurrence. We will also provide advice to help patients maintain a good quality of life during and after their treatment, providing helpful resources to help them get back on their feet both physically and mentally.

Throughout the pages of this book, you will encounter inspiring stories of people who have lived with cancer. These stories reflect the diversity of cancer patient experiences, from diagnosis to recovery and survival.

You will meet patients who were diagnosed at an early stage of the disease through regular screening and who were able to benefit from early and effective treatment. You will also hear testimonials from patients who overcame difficult obstacles, such as significant treatment side effects, and were able to return to a normal life after their treatment.

Also, you will find out how cancer research has progressed over the years and how it continues to develop. You will learn how healthcare professionals are working to improve existing treatments and develop new treatments for different forms of cancer.

The purpose of this book is to provide useful and practical information for cancer patients, as well as their families and friends. We hope this book will help you better understand cancer and its treatments, and help you make informed decisions about your health.

Finally, we would like to emphasize the importance of cancer prevention. Some forms of cancer can be prevented by adopting a healthy lifestyle, avoiding known risk factors, such as smoking, excessive alcohol consumption, exposure to cancer-causing chemicals, etc.

In conclusion, we hope you find this practical guide to cancer symptoms, causes and treatments helpful and informative. We hope this will give you a better understanding of this complex disease and help you navigate through the different stages of diagnosis and treatment. Together, we can continue to fight cancer and give cancer patients a chance for recovery and survival.

Chapter 1: Understanding cancers

Cancer is a complex and often difficult disease to understand. In this chapter we will explore the basics of cancer biology and what happens in the body when cancer develops.

I.   What is cancer?

Cancer is a disease in which abnormal cells grow out of control and invade surrounding tissue. These abnormal cells can also spread to other parts of the body, which is called metastasis.

Cancer can develop in almost every organ and tissue in our body. The most common types of cancer are breast cancer, lung cancer, prostate cancer, colon cancer, and skin cancer. However, there are many other less common types of cancer.

II.   How do cancers form?

First of all, it is important to understand that cancer does not involve a single disease, but rather a family of diseases which manifest themselves in different ways. Cells in our body are constantly dividing and multiplying to replace damaged or dead cells. However, sometimes these cells can start dividing uncontrollably and form a tumor.

A tumor can be benign or malignant. A benign tumor is a mass of cells that does not spread to other parts of the body and is not considered cancer. However, a malignant tumor is a group of cancer cells that can spread to other parts of the body and invade healthy tissue. Cancer can develop in almost every organ and tissue in our body.

Most cancers are the result of genetic mutations that affect cell growth and division. These mutations can be inherited or can occur during a person's lifetime due to exposure to risk factors such as smoking, prolonged exposure to radiation, unhealthy diet, etc.

It is important to note that everyone has genetic mutations, but not all of these mutations lead to cancer. Cells in our body have built-in mechanisms to detect and repair genetic errors that occur during normal cell division.

However, when these repair mechanisms fail, it can lead to genetic mutations that can cause cancer.

It is also important to understand that cancer is a constantly evolving process. Cancer cells can mutate and change over time, which can make the cancer more aggressive and harder to treat. This is why early diagnosis is so important, because the earlier the cancer is diagnosed, the easier it is to treat.

Finally, it is important to understand that cancer is not contagious. Cancer cells are abnormal cells that grow in our own body and cannot be passed from person to person.

III.   The different types of cancer

Cancer is not a single disease, but rather a collection of over 200 different diseases, so it is difficult to talk about cancer without understanding the specific type of cancer a person has. There are several ways to name and classify tumors, including by point of origin (cell, tissue, area), tumor grade, stage, DNA profile, and more. Knowing more about each of them can help you better understand the type of cancer you have and what it means for your journey.

1. Primary vs metastatic

An often confusing point in the discussion of cancer types occurs when a cancer spreads (metastasizes) to another area of the body. When a cancer spreads, it is named after the type of cancer cell or organ in which it started, not the area of the body where it spreads. It is primary cancer.

For example, if breast cancer starts in the breast and later spreads to the lung, it would not be called lung cancer. Instead, it would be called primary metastatic breast cancer of the lungs.

Rarely, doctors are unable to determine where a cancer started, only to find signs of cancer where it has spread. This is called cancer of unknown primary or cancer of unknown origin with metastases where the cancer is found.

2. By cell or tissue type

Many cancers are named after the type of cells in which the cancer begins. For example, you may have been told you have kidney cancer, but kidney cancers can differ greatly depending on the type of kidney cell in which these tumors start. There are six main types of cancer depending on the type of cell:

Carcinomas
Sarcomas
myeloma
Leukemias
Lymphomas
Mixed types (including blastomas)
Tumors may also be called "solid" or blood-related tumors. Blood-related cancers include leukemias, lymphomas, and myelomas, while solid cancers include all other cancers.

a) CARCINOMAS

Carcinoma is the most common type of cellular cancer, accounting for 80% to 90% of cancers. These cancers arise in cells called epithelial cells. Epithelial cells include skin cells and those that line body cavities and covering organs. Carcinomas can be divided into:

Adenocarcinomas: Adenocarcinomas start in gland cells that produce fluids, such as breast milk.

Squamous cell carcinomas: Examples of squamous cells include those in the upper layer of the skin, upper esophagus and airways, and lower cervix and vagina.

Basal cell carcinoma : Basal cells are found only in the skin and are the deepest layer of skin cells.

Transitional cell carcinomas: Transitional cells are "elastic" epithelial cells found in the bladder and parts of the kidney.

In addition to these more specific cell types, carcinomas can be named based on their location. For example, breast carcinomas that arise in the light ducts are called ductal carcinomas , while those that arise in the lobules are considered lobular carcinomas.

Carcinomas are the only types of cancer cells that have a non-invasive phase and, therefore, are the only cancers that are screened for regularly. Tumors that are still "contained" and have not spread through the basement membrane are called carcinoma in situ or CIN. Cancer detected at this early and pre-invasive stage should, in theory, be completely cured by ablation.

b) SARCOMA

Sarcomas are tumors of the bones and soft tissues of the body that are made up of cells called mesenchymal cells. These include tumors of bones, muscles (skeletal and smooth muscles), tendons, ligaments, cartilage, blood vessels, nerves, synovial tissues (joint tissues) and fatty tissues. Here are some examples of sarcomas:

Osteosarcoma (bone tumors)
Chondrosarcoma (cartilaginous tumors)
Liposarcoma (adipose tissue tumors)
Rhabdomyosarcoma (skeletal muscle tumors)
Leiomyosarcoma (smooth muscle tumors)
Angiosarcoma (blood vessel tumours)
Mesothelioma (tumors of the mesothelium , tissues

lining the chest and abdominal cavities)
Fibrosarcoma (fibrous tissue tumors)
Glioma and astrocytoma (connective tissue cells in the brain)

c) MYELOMA

Myeloma, also called multiple myeloma, is a cancer of immune system cells called plasma cells. Plasma cells are the cells that produce antibodies.

d) LEUKEMIA

Leukemias are tumors of blood cells and arise from the bone marrow. Among blood cancers, leukemias are considered "liquid tumors" unlike myeloma and lymphomas because they involve cells circulating in the blood, often treated as solid tumors that have spread. Here are some examples :

Lymphocytic leukemias: These are tumors of white blood cells called lymphocytes.
Myelocytic leukemias : These are tumors of mature or immature cells called myelocytes, such as neutrophils.
Lymphocytic and myelocytic leukemias have forms that progress quickly (acute) and forms that take longer to develop (chronic).

e) LYMPHOMA

Lymphomas are cancers that arise from cells of the immune system. These tumors can arise in the lymph nodes or from extranodal sites such as the spleen, stomach, or testicles. These are divided into:

Hodgkin's lymphoma

Non-Hodgkin lymphoma

3. MIXED TYPES

It is not uncommon for a cancer to show characteristics of more than one type of tissue. Cancer cells differ from normal cells in many ways, one of which is called differentiation.

Some types of cancer may closely resemble the normal cells in which they arise (these are called well-differentiated tumors), yet others may bear little resemblance to them (you may see the term undifferentiated on a pathology report).

Moreover, most cancers are heterogeneous. This means that cells in one part of a tumor can be very different from cells in another part of a tumor. For example, lung cancer may have cells that look like adenocarcinoma and others that look like squamous cell carcinoma. This would be described in a pathology report as having adenosquamous features .

Blablastomas are a type that is sometimes separated from others. These are tumors that occur in embryonic cells – cells that have not yet chosen a path to becoming epithelial cells or mesenchymal cells.

4. WHAT'S IN A NAME?

In general, cancerous tumors usually include the name of the particular cell type in which they started, followed by "sarcoma". For example, a benign bone tumor might be called an osteoma , but a malignant tumor an osteosarcoma .

5. BY BODY PART / SYSTEM

Tumors are also often separate from the organs or organ systems in which they arise.

a) Central nervous system tumors

Central nervous system tumors include those that arise from tissues in the brain or spinal cord. Tumors that spread to the brain are not considered brain tumors, but rather brain metastases and are much more common than primary brain tumors.

Tumors that commonly spread to the brain include lung cancer, breast cancer, and melanoma. Unlike tumors in other areas of the body, brain tumors often do not spread outside the brain.

Overall, the incidence of brain cancer has increased in recent years.

b) Head and neck cancer

Head and neck cancers can affect any area of the head and neck, from the tongue to the vocal cords. In the past, these cancers were most often seen in people who were both heavy drinkers and smokers. In recent years, however, the human papillomavirus (HPV) has become a major cause of these cancers, with nearly 10,000 people developing HPV-related head and neck cancers each year in the United States alone.

Two of these types of cancer are:

- Oral cancer: About 60-70% of all head and neck cancers are oral cancers, which can affect the mouth, tongue, tonsils, throat (pharynx), and nasal passages.
- Cancer of the larynx (cancer of the vocal cords)

c) Breast cancer

Many people know that breast cancer is an all too common cancer in women, but it is important to point out that men also get breast cancer. About 1 in 100 breast cancers occurs in men. The most common type of breast cancer is ductal carcinoma .

Because most breast cancers are carcinomas, they can sometimes be detected before they become invasive. This is considered carcinoma in situ or stage 0 breast cancer . Stages 1 through 4 of breast cancer are invasive stages of the disease. You may hear these more specific names:

ductal carcinoma in situ (DCIS) and lobular carcinoma in situ (LCIS): Carcinoma in situ is the first stage in which breast cancer can be detected and is considered stage 0. These tumors have not yet penetrated through the basement membrane and are considered non-invasive. They are detected most often when a biopsy is performed for an abnormality on a screening mammogram.

- Invasive (invasive) breast cancer (ductal and lobular): Once breast cancer penetrates through the basement membrane, it is considered invasive.

- Inflammatory breast cancer: Unlike other breast cancers, inflammatory breast cancer does not usually present as a lump. On the contrary, the early stages of the disease look like redness and a rash on the breast.
- Breast cancer in men: When breast cancer occurs in men, it is more likely to have a genetic component. A family history of breast cancer should stimulate a discussion with your doctor.

It can be scary to hear that you have "invasive" cancer, but that doesn't mean your cancer has spread. Stage 1 is also indicated in this way based on the appearance of the tumor under the microscope.

d) Respiratory tumors

Lung and bronchus cancers are the leading cause of cancer death for men and women in the United States. Although smoking is a risk factor for these diseases, lung cancer also occurs in non-smokers. In fact, lung cancer in these people is the sixth leading cause of cancer death in the United States.

Lung cancer is decreasing overall, probably due to a decrease in smoking. But it's on the rise among young adults, especially young women who never smoke. The reason is not understood at this time. Types you might hear about include:

Non-small cell lung cancer: Subtypes of non-small cell

lung cancer (responsible for approximately 80-85% of lung cancers) include adenocarcinoma of the lung, squamous cell carcinoma of the lungs, and lung cancer. large cell lung.

Small cell lung cancer: Small cell lung cancer accounts for about 15% of lung cancers and is more likely to occur in people who have smoked.

Mesothelioma : Mesothelioma is cancer of the pleural mesotheliolium , the lining surrounding the lungs. It is strongly linked to exposure to asbestos.

e) Digestive system tumors

Digestive tract cancers can occur anywhere from the mouth to the anus. Most of these tumors are adenocarcinomas, with squamous cell carcinomas occurring in the upper esophagus and the furthest part of the anus. Types include:

Esophageal cancer: The most common form of esophageal cancer has changed in recent years. While esophageal squamous cell cancer (often linked to smoking and alcohol consumption) was once the most common form of the disease, it has been overtaken by esophageal adenocarcinoma (often linked to acid reflux from long time).

Stomach cancer: Stomach cancer is rare in the United States, but it is a common type of cancer worldwide.

Pancreatic cancer: Pancreatic cancer is less common than some other cancers, but it is the fourth most common cause of cancer-related death in both men and women. It is most often diagnosed in the later stages of the disease, when surgery is unfortunately no longer possible.

Liver cancer: Metastatic liver cancer is much more common than primary liver cancer. Risk factors for liver cancer include alcohol abuse and chronic hepatitis B or C infections.

Colon cancer: Colon cancer is often called colorectal cancer and includes cancers of the rectum and upper colon. It is the third leading cause of cancer death in both men and women.

Cancer: Cancer differs from colon cancer in treatments and causes. HPV infection now causes most cancers.

f) Urinary system tumors

The genitourinary system involves the kidneys, the bladder, the tubes connecting the kidneys and the bladder (called the ureters), and the urethra (the bladder passage). This system also includes structures such as the prostate. Types include:

Kidney cancer: The most common types of kidney cancer include renal cell carcinoma (about 90% of cases), transitional cell carcinoma, and Wilms tumor in children.

Bladder cancer: About half of bladder cancers are caused by exposure to tobacco, and those who work with dyes and paints are also at higher risk.

Prostate cancer: The prostate is the second leading cause of cancer death in men, but now has a very high five-year survival rate.

g) Tumors of the reproductive system

Tumors of the reproductive organs can occur in both men and women. Ovarian cancer is the fifth most

common cause of cancer death in women and
although it can be treated at an early stage, it is often
diagnosed when it has already spread. Types include:

Testicular cancer
Ovarian cancer (including germ cell cancers)
Uterine cancer (also called endometrial cancer)
Fallopian tube cancer
Cervical cancer

h) Endocrine cancer

The endocrine system is a series of glands that
produce hormones and as such can show symptoms
of either overproduction or underproduction of these
hormones. Most endocrine cancers, with the
exception of thyroid cancer, are quite rare. A
combination of multiple endocrine tumors can run in
families and is called multiple endocrine neoplasia, or
MEN.

The incidence of thyroid cancer is increasing in the
United States more than any other cancer.
Fortunately, the survival rate for many of these
cancers is high.

i) Bone and soft tissue tumors

Unlike primary bone and soft tissue tumors, which
are rare, metastatic cancer to bone is common. Bone
cancer, primary or metastatic, often presents with
symptoms of pain or a pathological fracture, a
fracture that occurs in a bone weakened by the
presence of a tumor. Types include:

Kaposi's sarcoma: Kaposi's sarcoma is a soft tissue cancer often seen in people living with HIV/AIDS. Ewing's sarcoma: Ewing's sarcoma is a bone cancer that mainly affects children.

j) Blood-related cancers

Blood-related cancers include both those involving blood cells and those involving solid tissues of the immune system, such as the lymph nodes. Risk factors for blood-related cancers differ somewhat from solid cancers in that environmental exposure and viruses (such as Epstein-Barr virus, which causes mononucleosis) play an important role. These are the most common tumors in children.

Blood-related cancers include:

Hodgkin's lymphoma
Non-Hodgkin lymphoma
lymphoblastic leukemia
Chronic lymphocytic leukemia
Acute myeloid leukemia
Chronic myeloid leukemia
Myeloma

k) Skin cancer

Skin cancers are often divided into two main groups: melanoma and non-melanoma. While non-melanoma skin cancers are much more common, melanomas are responsible for the majority of skin cancer deaths.

Here are some examples of skin cancers:

- Basal cell carcinoma
- Squamous cell carcinoma of the skin

6. OTHER CLASSIFICATION METHODS

In addition to grouping tumors in the above way, tumors are often classified by:

a) Tumor grade:

Grade is a measure of how aggressive a tumor is. A grade 1 tumor is less aggressive and the cells may look very similar to the normal cells in which the cancer started. A grade 3 tumor, on the other hand, is usually more aggressive and the cells look very different from normal cells.

b) Tumor stage:

Tumors are organized in different ways, but many are assigned a number between 1 and 4, with 4 representing the most advanced stage of the cancer.

c) Non-hereditary cancer vs hereditary cancer:

Some types of cancer are called hereditary tumors. For example, about 5-10% of breast cancers are defined as such: there is a lot of overlap, and genetics plays a role in many cancers.

d) DNA/molecular profiles:

As our understanding of genetics improves, cancers are more frequently classified based on their genetic profile. For example, some lung cancers have EGFR mutations, while others have ALK rearrangements.

If you are diagnosed with a rare cancer, it may be worth seeking a second opinion from one of the major cancer centers designated by the National Cancer Institute. These larger centers are more likely to have oncologists on staff who have a particular interest in less common, but no less important, cancers.

Chapter 2 : Cancer risk factors

In general, it is not possible to know exactly why one person has cancer and another does not. But research has indicated that certain risk factors can increase a person's risk of cancer. (There are also certain factors that are linked to a lower risk of cancer. These factors are sometimes called protective factors.)

IV.   Risk factors

Risk factors for cancer include exposure to chemicals or other substances, as well as certain behaviors. They also include things people can't control, like age and family history.

A family history of certain cancers can be a sign of a possible hereditary cancer syndrome.

Most cancer risk factors (and protective factors) are initially identified in epidemiological studies. In these studies, scientists look at large groups of people and compare people with cancer to those without.

These studies can show that people who develop cancer are more or less likely to behave in certain ways or have been exposed to certain substances than people who do not have cancer.

Such studies, by themselves, cannot prove that a behavior or substance causes cancer. For example, the finding could be the result of chance, or the true risk factor could be other than the suspected risk factor.
But findings like this sometimes attract media attention, which can lead to misconceptions about how cancer starts and how it spreads.

When numerous studies indicate that there is a similar association between a possible risk factor and an increased risk of cancer, and when there is a possible mechanism that explains how the risk factor might actually cause cancer, scientists will be more confident in the relationship between the two.

The list below includes known or suspected cancer risk factors that have been most studied. Although some of these risk factors can be avoided; Others, like aging, cannot be avoided.
By limiting exposure to preventable risk factors, you can reduce your risk of developing certain cancers.

1. Alcohol

Drinking alcohol can increase your risk of mouth, throat, esophagus, larynx, liver and breast cancer. The more you drink, the greater your risk . The risk of cancer is much higher for those who drink alcohol and also use tobacco.

Doctors advise those who drink to drink in

moderation. The federal government's Dietary Guidelines for Americans define moderate alcohol consumption for women, up to one drink a day; for men up to two glasses a day.

Certain substances in red wine, such as resveratrol , have been suggested to have anti-cancer properties. However, there is no evidence that drinking red wine reduces the risk of cancer.

2. Diet

Many studies have examined the possibility that specific food components or nutrients are associated with an increased or decreased risk of cancer. Studies of cancer cells in the laboratory and in animal models sometimes provide evidence that isolated chemical compounds may be carcinogenic (or have anti-cancer activity).

But, with few exceptions, studies in human populations have yet to definitively show that any dietary component causes or protects against cancer. Sometimes the results of epidemiological studies comparing diets with those of people with and without cancer have indicated that people with and without cancer differ in their consumption of a particular component of the diet.

However, these results only indicate that the dietary component is associated with a change in cancer risk, not that the dietary component is responsible or causes the change in risk. For example, participants with or without cancer may differ in ways other than their diet, and it is possible that another difference is responsible for the difference in cancer.

When an epidemiological study demonstrates that a food component is associated with a lower risk of cancer, a randomized study can be carried out to test this possibility. Random assignment ensures that any difference between people who have a high or low intake of a nutrient is due to the nutrient itself rather than other differences that were not detected. (For ethical reasons, randomized studies are generally not performed when there is evidence that a food component may be associated with an increased risk of cancer.

Scientists have studied many additives, nutrients, and other food components to look for possible associations with cancer risk. It is :

Although red wine has been suspected of reducing cancer risk, there is no scientific evidence for such an association. Also, alcohol is known to cause cancer. Excessive or regular alcohol consumption increases the risk of cancers of the oral cavity (excluding the lips), pharynx (throat), larynx, esophagus, liver, breast, colon and throat. rectum. The risk of cancer increases with the amount of alcohol a person drinks. To find out more, consult the fact sheet Alcohol and the risk of cancer

Antioxidants are chemical compounds that block the activity of other chemical compounds called free radicals that can damage cells. Laboratory and animal research has shown that exogenous antioxidants can help prevent free radical damage associated with cancer formation, but human research has not convincingly shown that taking antioxidant supplements may help reduce the risk of developing cancer or dying from cancer.

Some studies have even shown an increased risk of certain cancers. For more information, see the Antioxidants and Cancer Prevention fact sheet.

Studies have been conducted on the safety of several artificial sweeteners, such as saccharin, aspartame, acesulfame potassium , sucralose , neotame , and cyclamate. There is no clear evidence to suggest that artificial sweeteners commercially available in the United States are associated with cancer risk in humans. For more information, see the fact sheet Artificial Sweeteners and Cancer.

Calcium is an essential dietary mineral that can be obtained from foods and dietary supplements. Research results generally support the relationship between high calcium intake and a reduced risk of colorectal cancer, but study results have not always been consistent. It is unclear whether there is a link between high calcium intake and a reduced risk of other cancers such as breast and ovarian cancer. Some research suggests that a high calcium intake may increase the risk of prostate cancer.

To learn more, see the fact sheet Calcium and Cancer Prevention: Strength and Limits of Scientific Evidence.

Certain chemical compounds, called heterocyclic amines (HCAs) and polycyclic aromatic hydrocarbons (PAHs), are formed in muscle meat, including beef, pork, fish and poultry, when cooked using methods at high temperature. Exposure to high concentrations of heterocyclic amines and polycyclic aromatic hydrocarbons can cause cancer in animals; However, it is unclear whether such exposure causes cancer in humans. For more information, see the fact sheet Meat cooked at high temperatures and the risk of cancer.

Cruciferous vegetables contain chemicals called glucosinolates , which are broken down into several chemical compounds that are being studied for their possible anti-cancer effects. Some of these compounds have shown anti-cancer effects in cells and animals, but the results of human studies have not been as clear. For more information, see the Cruciferous Plants and Cancer Prevention fact sheet.

Fluoride in water helps prevent tooth decay and even reverses the process of tooth decay. Numerous studies, both in humans and in animals, have shown that there is no link between fluoridated water and the risk of cancer. For more information, see the Fluoridated Water fact sheet.

Tea contains chemical compounds of polyphenols, especially catechins, which are antioxidants. The results of epidemiological studies that have examined the relationship between tea consumption and cancer risk have been inconclusive. Few clinical studies have been conducted on tea drinking and cancer prevention and the results have been inconclusive. For more information, see the Tea and Cancer Prevention Fact Sheet.

Vitamin D helps the body use calcium and phosphorus to build strong bones and teeth. It is mainly obtained by exposing the skin to sunlight, but can also be obtained from certain foods and dietary supplements.

Human epidemiological studies have indicated that higher vitamin D intake or higher vitamin D blood levels may be associated with lower risks of colorectal cancer, but results from randomized studies have been inconclusive. For more information, see the Vitamin D and cancer prevention fact sheet.

3. Age

Old age is the most important risk factor for cancer in general and many cancers in particular. The cancer incidence rate (new cases) increases with age.

According to the most recent statistical data from the National Cancer Institute (NCI) Surveillance, Epidemiology, and End Results (SEER) Program, the median age at diagnosis of cancer is 66 years. That is, half of cancer cases are diagnosed in people under 66 and the other half in people over 62. A similar trend is seen in many common cancers. For example, the median age at diagnosis is 67 for breast cancer, 71 for colorectal cancer, 66 for lung cancer, and <> years for prostate cancer.

But it is possible to be diagnosed with cancer at any age. For example, bone cancer is most often diagnosed in children under the age of 20 (children and adolescents), and about 25% of cases occur in this age group. Furthermore, 12% of cases of brain cancer and other cancers of the nervous system are diagnosed in children and adolescents, while only 1% of all cancers are diagnosed in this age group.

4. infectious germs

Certain infectious germs, including viruses, bacteria and parasites, can cause cancer or increase the risk of cancer. Some viruses can disrupt signals that normally control cell growth and proliferation. Also, some infections weaken the immune system, making the body less able to fight off other carcinogenic infections. And some viruses, bacteria, and parasites also cause chronic inflammation that can lead to cancer.

Most viruses that are linked to an increased risk of cancer can be passed from person to person through blood or other body fluids.

5. Hormone

Estrogens, a group of female sex hormones, are known to be carcinogenic to humans. Although these hormones have essential physiological functions in both women and men, they have also been linked to an increased risk of certain cancers.

For example, taking combination hormone therapy during menopause (estrogen plus progestin, which is a synthetic form of the female hormone progesterone) may increase a woman's risk of breast cancer. Postmenopausal hormone therapy with estrogen alone increases the risk of endometrial cancer and is only used in women who have had a hysterectomy.

A woman considering menopausal hormone therapy should talk to her doctor about the possible risks and benefits of menopause.

Studies have also indicated that a woman's risk of developing breast cancer is related to the estrogen and progesterone produced by her ovaries (called endogenous estrogen and progesterone). Long-term exposure or high levels of these hormones have been linked to an increased risk of breast cancer. Increased exposure may be caused by starting menstruation at a younger age, reaching menopause at a later age, being older when first pregnancy occurs, and never having gave birth. Conversely, childbirth is a protective factor in breast cancer.

6. Chronic inflammation

Inflammation is a normal physiological response that causes injured tissue to heal. An inflammatory process begins when chemical compounds are released from damaged tissues.

In response, white blood cells produce substances that cause cells to divide and grow to rebuild tissue to help repair injuries. Once the wound has healed, the inflammatory process will end.

In chronic inflammation, the inflammatory process may start even when there is no injury and not end when it should. It is not always clear why the inflammation continues. Chronic inflammation can be caused by infections that don't go away, abnormal immune reactions to normal tissues, or conditions like obesity.

Over time, chronic inflammation can cause DNA damage and lead to cancer. For example, people with chronic inflammatory bowel diseases, such as ulcerative colitis and Crohn 's disease , have an increased risk of colon cancer.

7. Immunosuppression

Many people who receive an organ transplant take drugs to suppress the immune system so that the body does not reject the organ.

These "immunosuppressive" drugs make the immune system less able to detect and kill cancer cells or fight cancer-causing infections. HIV infection also weakens the immune system and increases the risk of certain cancers.

Research has indicated that transplant recipients have increased risks of many different cancers. Some of these cancers are caused by infectious germs while others are not.

The four most common cancers in transplant recipients that occur more frequently in these individuals than in the general population are non-Hodgkin's lymphoma (NHL) and cancers of the lung, kidney and liver.

8. Sunlight

The sun, sunlamps and tanning beds or rooms emit ultraviolet (UV) rays. Exposure to UV rays causes premature skin aging and damage that can lead to skin cancer.

People of all ages and skin tones should limit their time in the sun. In particular, avoid being in the sun between 10 a.m. and 4 a.m. Also, do not be exposed to other sources of UV radiation, such as tanning beds.

Keep in mind that UV rays reflect (bounce) off sand, water, snow and ice and pass through the windshield and car windows. Although skin cancer is more common in lighter-skinned people, skin cancer occurs in people with any skin tone, even if they have dark skin.

9. Obesity

People who are obese may have an increased risk of several types of cancer, including cancers of the breast (in postmenopausal women), colon, rectum, endometrium (lining of the uterus), esophagus, kidney, pancreas and gallbladder.

Conversely, healthy eating, physical activity and maintaining a healthy weight can reduce the risk of certain cancers. These healthy behaviors are also important for reducing the risk of other diseases, such as heart disease, type 2 diabetes, and high blood pressure.

10. Radiation

Radiation of certain wavelengths, called ionizing radiation, has enough energy to damage DNA and cause cancer. Ionizing radiation includes radon, x-rays, gamma rays, and other forms of high-energy radiation. Low-energy, non-ionizing forms of radiation, such as visible light and cell phone energy, have not caused cancer in people.

Substances in the environment that cause cancer

11. Tobacco

Tobacco is the leading cause of cancer and cancer death. People who use tobacco products or who are regularly near environmental tobacco smoke (also called second-hand smoke) have an increased risk of cancer because tobacco products and second-hand smoke contain many chemicals that damage the body. DNA.

Smoking causes many types of cancer, including cancer of the lung, larynx, mouth, esophagus, throat, bladder, kidney, liver, stomach, pancreas, colon and rectum, and cervix or cervix, as well as acute myeloid leukemia. People who use smokeless tobacco (snuff or chewing tobacco) are at increased risk of cancer of the mouth, esophagus and pancreas.

There is no harmless degree in tobacco use. People who use any type of tobacco product are urged to stop using it.
People who quit smoking, regardless of their age, have a substantial gain in life expectancy compared to those who continue to smoke. In addition, quitting smoking at the time of a cancer diagnosis reduces the risk of death.

12. Genetic changes and cancer

Cancer is a genetic disease, which means cancer is caused by certain changes in the genes that control how our cells work, specifically how they grow and divide.

Genes carry the instructions for making proteins, which do much of the work in our cells. Certain genetic changes can cause cells to escape normal growth controls and become cancerous.

For example, some carcinogenic genetic changes increase the production of a protein that makes cells grow. Others result in the production of a disfigured, and therefore non-functional, form of a protein that would normally repair cellular damage.

Genetic changes that promote cancer can be inherited from our parents if the changes are present in germ cells, which are the body's reproductive cells (eggs and sperm). These types of changes, called germline changes, are found in each of the cells of the offspring.

Carcinogenic genetic changes can also be acquired during a person's lifetime, as a result of DNA errors that occur when cells divide or exposure to DNA-damaging carcinogens, such as as certain chemicals in tobacco smoke, or radiation, such as ultraviolet rays from the sun. Genetic changes that occur after conception are called somatic (or acquired) changes.

There are many types of DNA changes. Some changes only affect a single unit of DNA, called a nucleotide. A nucleotide can be replaced by another, or it can be completely absent. Other changes involve larger stretches of DNA and may include rearrangements, deletions, or duplications of long stretches of DNA.

Sometimes the changes are not in the precise DNA sequence. For example, adding or removing chemical marks, called epigenetic modifications , to DNA can influence how the gene is "expressed", i.e. if and how much messenger RNA is produced . (The messenger RNA is translated, in turn, to produce the proteins encoded by the DNA.)

In general, cancer cells have more genetic changes than normal cells. However, each person's cancer has a unique combination of genetic alterations. Some of these changes may be consequences of the cancer and not its causes. As the cancer continues to grow, other changes will occur. Even within the same tumor, cancer cells can have different genetic changes.

Chapter 3: Risk factors specific to certain cancers

A risk factor is anything that increases or decreases a person's chance of suffering from a disease. Although doctors cannot explain why one person develops the disease and another does not, researchers have identified specific factors that increase a person's chance of developing certain types of cancer.

Cancer risk factors can be divided into four groups:

Behavioral risk factors refer to things you do, such as smoking, drinking alcohol, using tanning beds, eating unhealthy foods, being overweight, and not getting enough exercise.

Environmental risk factors include things in the environment around you, such as UV rays, exposure to second-hand smoke, pollution, pesticides, and other toxins.

Biological risk factors are physical characteristics, such as gender, race or ethnicity, age, and skin color.
Hereditary risk factors are linked to specific genetic mutations inherited from parents. You are more likely to get cancer if you inherit one of these genetic mutations.

Most behavioral and environmental cancer risk factors are preventable. Biological and hereditary risk factors are unavoidable, but it's important to be aware of them so you can discuss them with your doctor and get tested for cancer if needed.

I. What are the risk factors for different types of cancer?

1. Breast cancer

Age: Most cases occur in women 50 and older
Family history of breast or ovarian cancer before menopause (mother, sister or daughter)

Abnormal breast biopsy results
Ductal or lobular carcinoma in situ or atypical hyperplasia
First menstruation before the age of 12
Menopause after 55
Never have been pregnant or had the first child after the age of 30
High educational and socio-economic level
Women in this group tend to have fewer children
Obesity or weight gain after menopause
Hormonal treatment
Inherited mutations in the BRCA1 or BRCA2 genes
Other suspected risk factors include:
high fat diet
Physical inactivity
Drink more than one alcoholic drink per day
Use of oral contraceptives

2. Cervical cancer

First sexual intercourse at an early age
Multiple sexual partners (of the woman or her partner)
Smoking
Race: More cases occur in black or Latino women
Human papillomavirus (HPV) infection
Exposure to diethylstilbestrol (DES) before birth
HIV infection
Weakened immune system due to organ transplant, chemotherapy, or chronic steroid use

3. Colorectal cancer

Age: more common in people over 50
Family or personal history of colorectal cancer (especially in father, mother or sibling)
Family or personal history of adenomatous polyps (especially in father, mother, or sibling)
Personal history of inflammatory bowel disease
Diet high in fat (especially red meat)
Diet low in fiber, fruits and vegetables
Physical inactivity
Smoking
Alcohol consumption
Obesity

4. Endometrial cancer (also called uterine cancer)

Aging
Increased estrogen exposure
First menstruation before the age of 12
Menopause after 55
Hormonal treatment without the use of progestins
Never have been pregnant
History of infertility
Personal history of hereditary nonpolyposis colon cancer
Obesity
Use of tamoxifen

5. Lung cancer

Smoking in the form of cigarettes, cigars or pipes
Family or personal history of lung cancer
Recurring exposure to:
Radon or asbestos (especially in smokers)
Radiation
Arsenic
Atmospheric pollution
Tobacco smoke (passive exposure)
Lung diseases such as tuberculosis (TB)

6. Ovarian cancer

Age: more common in women over 50
Family history of ovarian cancer (mother, daughter, sister, grandmother or aunt)
Inherited mutations in the BRCA1 or BRCA2 genes
Northern European or Ashkenazi Jewish ancestry
Never have been pregnant
Other suspected risk factors include:
Fertility drugs
Exposure to talcum powder
Hormone replacement therapy
Obesity

7. Prostate cancer

Age: Men 50 and older are more at risk
Family history of prostate cancer (especially father, sibling, or child)
Race: Incidence in black males is almost double that seen in white males
Diet high in saturated fat and low in fruits and

vegetables

8. Skin cancer

Exposure to ultraviolet (UV) rays from the sun or use of tanning beds
Clear complexion
Family history, especially melanoma
Living in southern countries or close to the so-called "sun belt" (at latitudes of $\pm 35°$ from the equator)
Live in a sunny climate
Occupational exposure to:
Mineral tar
pitch
Creosote
Arsenic
Radio

II.   How to reduce your cancer risk

Cancer is a disease that can arise due to different factors. Although there is no 100% effective prevention method, lifestyle improvements can help reduce the risk of disease. Check out some tips.

Cancer is a disease caused by changes in the genes that control the growth and division of cells in the body. It can occur almost anywhere on the body and, in fact, sometimes affects multiple organs at the same time.

Today there is a lot of speculation on this issue, but

there is no specific information on what can reduce the risk of suffering from the disease, or what foods and habits we should change to avoid its occurrence. . However, it is suggested that certain lifestyle changes could have an impact on making us more susceptible to developing the disease or avoiding it. Therefore, it is important to have a balanced diet, adopt healthy habits, do regular physical activity, among others.

Here are some helpful tips that can help you reduce your risk of cancer. You must bear in mind that, since it is a disease of multifactorial origin, these habits are not entirely decisive in preventing its development.

1. Avoid exposure to carcinogens

Certain substances, such as asbestos, benzene, glyphosate, among others, could be linked to an increased risk of developing cancer. In this regard, a review of molecular medicine reports suggests that prolonged exposure to these compounds impairs body functions, which contributes to the onset of disease.

Therefore, it is very important to know the risks of these substances and to learn how to identify them to avoid contact with them. Below we detail what are its main characteristics and possible risks, according to the aforementioned review.

a) Asbestos

This fiber is one of the most polluting products for the environment and has been used for years, for its thermal properties, for the construction of buildings and roads.

Although the studies are not yet conclusive as to their influence on the development of the disease, there are several indications that the inhalation of these fibers could be responsible for the development of certain types of cancer, such as lung cancer.

b) Benzene

Benzene is an aromatic hydrocarbon used for industrial purposes and present in the air, mainly through the smoke given off by wood, gasoline and tobacco.

The World Health Organization (WHO) warns that exposure to this substance can cause several diseases, such as aplastic anemia and several types of cancer such as stomach, prostate and nose.

c) Glyphosate

Glyphosate is a herbicide used worldwide, for agricultural or domestic purposes, for the eradication and control of any pest.

Although studies are not conclusive, it is suggested that prolonged or regular exposure to its chemical compounds may influence the development of certain diseases, such as multiple sclerosis, asthma, diabetes, and Alzheimer's and Parkinsons.

2. Avoid tobacco to reduce the risk of cancer

Tobacco contains several substances that are

potentially harmful to health and can contribute to the onset of this disease. A study published in Oncotarget Journal mentions that it can compromise the health of different parts of the body, such as the mouth, larynx, bladder, cervix, among others.

This same study indicates that smoking is linked to at least 13 different types of cancer, including lung, bladder, kidney and pancreas.

It is important to remember that not only smokers, but also passive smoking are at risk. Second-hand smoke carries several harmful substances, as a person who accidentally inhales it can also develop cancer. Therefore, it is essential to avoid this bad habit in all its forms.

3. Decrease alcohol consumption

According to a review of studies published in Molecular Diversity Preservation International, the findings suggest that excessive alcohol consumption may increase the risk of several chronic non-communicable diseases, including breast and colon cancer. Therefore, it is essential to limit its consumption as much as possible.

4. Maintain a healthy diet

A healthy diet is basically one in which a good ratio is established between carbohydrates, proteins, fruits and vegetables, in addition to including fresh foods and avoiding those that are processed.

To this last group correspond industrial-type foods known as junk food or packaged foods. Therefore, the more natural the food, the more beneficial it will be for health.

A publication in American Family Physician , suggests that a healthy, balanced diet should include fruits and vegetables, fats, proteins, legumes, whole grains and nuts. It is recommended that fruits and vegetables occupy at least half of the plate. It is also essential to limit the consumption of added sugar to less than 10% of daily caloric intake.

5. Do physical activity every day

Exercise has proven to be a good ally when it comes to maintaining physical condition and helping to prevent certain diseases, ranging from overweight and stress to cancer. However, it should be remembered that not all organisms have the same physical capacity. Therefore, it is necessary to go to the doctor to establish an effective routine according to the needs of each person.

When it comes to cancer, a review published in the Canadian Medical Association suggests that a routine of moderate physical activity, lasting 30 to 60 minutes a day, helps reduce the risk of certain types of cancer, such as the colon and breast.

6. Use sunscreen

Skin cancer has become one of the most common,

and its main cause is the lack of protection when exposed to the sun. Therefore, it is very important to apply sunscreen every day, even when the day is cloudy or rainy.

Although sunlight is necessary for certain body functions, a study published in the European Journal of Cancer explains that frequent and prolonged exposure to sunlight affects an increased risk of skin cancer or melanoma.

According to this, it is best to avoid direct sun exposure, especially between 10 a.m. and 4 p.m. If there is no alternative, it is advisable to wear sunglasses and a wide-brimmed hat. It should also cover the skin as much as possible and stay in the shade.

7. Take care of your body weight

Maintaining a healthy weight is important when it comes to taking care of your health, as it not only decreases the risk of cardiovascular disease, diabetes and hypertension, but also the risk of suffering from different types of cancer.

A study published in Cancer Causes and Control warns that being overweight is directly linked to an increased risk of cancer of the colon, kidney, pancreas, endometrium and esophagus. On top of that, multiple tests show that it also increases the risk of leukemia, lymphoma, multiple myeloma, and liver and gallbladder cancers.

Chapter 4: the most common cancers and their symptoms

Globally, the most common cancers are lung and breast cancers, accounting for approximately 25% of all cancers diagnosed.

Below, we outline the cancers that had a higher incidence in 2018, marking the cases that were diagnosed that year.

I.   The most common cancers

1. Lung cancer

Lung cancer is the most common type of cancer and the one that causes the most deaths in the world. Smoking is the leading cause of lung cancer in both active and passive smokers.

However, it can also develop in people who have never smoked or lived with smokers; in which case the causes are not very clear.

Lung cancer does not usually cause symptoms in the early stages of its development, but occurs when the disease is more advanced. These symptoms are usually the following:

Cough (sometimes bloody)
Shortness of breath
Hoarseness
Chest pain
Weightloss
Bone and cranial pain

2. Breast cancer

Although it can occur in both sexes, breast cancer is much more common in women, being the type of cancer they are most often diagnosed with. Early detection of the tumor is essential to increase the survival rate.

The causes that lead to its development are not very clear, since it usually occurs due to a complex interaction between genetics and the environment.

It has been observed that there are risk factors related to hormones and lifestyle, although there are times when people with these risk factors never develop breast cancer and others without these factors, yes.

The most common symptoms of breast cancer are:

Breast mass
Morphological changes in the breast
Dimples in the breast
Nipple indentation
Peeling and crusting of the skin surrounding the nipple
Breast redness

3. Colorectal cancer

Colorectal cancer is a type of cancer that develops in the large intestine (colon) and can reach the anal rectum. It usually affects adults over the age of 50.

Doctors don't know exactly what causes this type of cancer, but it is known that there are certain risk factors that can increase the risk of developing it: older age, chronic inflammatory bowel conditions, family history, poor diets in fiber and high in fat, sedentary lifestyle, diabetes, obesity, smoking, alcohol...

The most common symptoms include:

Diarrhea
Constipation
Change in stool consistency
Rectal bleeding
Weightloss
Fatigue and weakness
Abdominal pain

4. Prostate cancer

This type of cancer occurs in the prostate, a gland present in men that produces seminal fluid, a means of nourishing and transporting sperm. Prostate cancer is one of the most common types of cancer in men.

Although they don't know the exact causes, doctors do know that there are certain risk factors : older age, race (it's more common in African-American men), obesity, and a family history.

Symptoms, which appear in advanced stages of the disease, are as follows:

blood in semen
erectile dysfunction
Difficulty urinating
Discomfort in the pelvic region
Bone pain

5. Skin cancer (other than melanoma)

Skin cancer usually develops in areas of the epidermis that are exposed to the sun, although it can also develop in areas where solar radiation does not affect. The "non-melanoma" group includes all skin cancers that occur without the formation of melanoma (about 280,000 cases of this type are reported each year).

The main cause of skin cancer is excessive exposure to the sun without protection, because the ultraviolet radiation causes damage in the cells, which makes them cancerous.
Be that as it may, there are other risk factors: having fair skin, the presence of moles on the skin, weakening of the immune system, family history, skin lesions, etc.

Although they vary greatly depending on the region of the body in which it develops, the most common symptoms of skin cancer are:

Development of ulcers
Brown lesions
Pieces of skin
bleeding moles
Itchy wounds

6. Stomach cancer

Stomach cancer starts in the mucus-producing cells that line the stomach, usually at the top of the stomach.

One of the main causes for the development of stomach cancer is gastroesophageal reflux disease and, to a lesser extent, smoking and obesity. It is also believed that a diet in which many salty and smoked foods and few fruits and vegetables are consumed can lead to the development of this type of cancer. There are also other risk factors: family history, bacterial infections, inflammation of the stomach, anemia...

The most common symptoms caused by stomach cancer are:

Fatigue
Bloated feeling
Quick satiety
Indigestion
Frequent vomiting
Slimming
Nausea
stomach pain
Heartburn

7. Liver cancer

Liver cancer starts in liver cells. One cause that leads to the development of the tumor is thought to be hepatitis, although it can also occur in previously healthy people, in which case the causes are not too clear.

However, there are risk factors: excessive alcohol consumption, cirrhosis, diabetes, exposure to aflatoxins, family history, etc.

Although it is asymptomatic in the early stages, the most common symptoms are:

Weightloss
Whitish stools
Weakness and fatigue
Loss of appetite
Yellowing of the skin
Abdominal pain
Nausea and vomiting

8. Esophageal cancer

Esophageal cancer, more common in men than women, develops in the cells that line the inside of the esophagus, which connects the throat to the stomach.

The causes are unclear, although there are risk factors: smoking, obesity, alcoholism, bile and/or gastroesophageal reflux, consumption of very hot drinks, diet low in fruits and vegetables, etc.

The most common symptoms of esophageal cancer are:

Difficulty swallowing
Weightloss
Chest pain
Burning of chest and stomach
Indigestion
Cough

9. Cervical cancer

Cervical cancer is the type of cancer that develops in the lower part of the uterus which connects to the vagina.

The main cause of developing cervical cancer is having an infection with the human papillomavirus (HPV), although not all women with HPV develop cancer. There are therefore other risk factors: smoking, weakening of the immune system, sexually transmitted infections, sexual intercourse at an early age, etc.

Symptoms appear at an advanced stage and are as follows:

Vaginal bleeding after sex
Discharge and bloody vaginal discharge
Pelvic pain
Pain during sex

10. Thyroid cancer

This type of cancer occurs in the thyroid, an endocrine gland that produces hormones responsible for regulating heart rate, body temperature, weight and blood pressure.

The causes that lead to its development are not clear, although it is known that there are risk factors: being a woman, being exposed to high levels of radiation and genetic syndromes.

The most common symptoms of thyroid cancer are:

bump in the neck
Voice changes

Difficulty swallowing
Pain in the throat
Swollen lymph nodes

11. Bladder cancer

Bladder cancer starts in the urothelial cells of the bladder, the organ in which urine is stored. It generally affects men more than women, and although it can appear at any time of life, it most often develops in old age.

The most common causes of bladder cancer are: smoking, exposure to high doses of radiation or chemical compounds, chronic bladder irritation and parasitic infections.

The most common symptoms associated with this type of cancer are:

Hematuria (presence of blood in the urine)
Polyuria (need to urinate several times a day)
Pelvic pain
Pain during urination
back pain

12. Non-Hodgkin lymphoma

Non-Hodgkin's lymphoma is a type of cancer that develops in the lymphatic system. It affects white blood cells, the cells responsible for the proper functioning of the immune system.

Doctors do not know exactly the causes that lead

these cells to become tumors, although it usually happens when the immune system is weakened, which can be given by different risk factors: consumption of immunosuppressive drugs, viral or bacterial infections , exposure to chemical substances, advanced age, etc.

The most common symptoms of this type of cancer are:

Weightloss
Fatigue
Abdominal pain
Swollen lymph nodes (neck, armpits or groin)
Fever
Night sweats
Cough
Shortness of breath
Chest pain

13. Pancreatic cancer

This type of cancer affects the cells of the pancreas, an organ responsible for secreting enzymes for digestion and hormones that regulate blood sugar levels.

Although the causes are not very clear, different risk factors have been determined that increase the chances of developing it: smoking, obesity, advanced age over 65, pancreatitis, diabetes, family history, etc.

Typical symptoms of pancreatic cancer are:

Abdominal pain
back pain
Diabetes
Blood clots
Fatigue
Jaundice (whitening of the skin)
Weightloss
Loss of appetite
Depression

14. Leukemia

Leukemia is a type of cancer that develops in the blood. There are many types of leukemia (some affect children and some affect adults) although in general all are characterized by affecting the functioning of white blood cells.

It is not known exactly what causes leukemia, although there are risk factors: smoking, exposure to chemical compounds, history of cancer treatment, genetic disorders and family history.

The most common symptoms associated with leukemia are:

Fever
Chills
Fatigue and weakness
Weightloss
Recurrent infections
Weakened immune system
Nosebleeds
Night sweats

Swollen lymph nodes
Appearance of bruises
Petechiae (red spots on the skin)
Bone pain

15. kidney cancer

Kidney cancer develops in kidney cells. The risk factors associated with this disease are: smoking, advanced age, obesity, hypertension, dialysis, exposure to chemical compounds, genetic disorders, family history, etc.

The most common symptoms of kidney cancer include:

Hematuria (blood in the urine)
Weightloss
Loss of appetite
Fatigue and weakness
Fever
back pain

16. endometrial cancer

Endometrial cancer is cancer that starts in the uterus, the organ in which fetal development occurs during pregnancy. This cancer is usually detected at an early stage because it causes abnormal vaginal bleeding.

Risk factors that increase the likelihood of endometrial cells becoming cancerous are: never having been pregnant, starting menstruation at an early age, old age, obesity, treatment of breast cancer with hormones and changes in the hormonal balance of a woman's body.

Symptoms, which appear in the early stages of the development of the disease, are:

Bleeding outside the menstrual season
Postmenopausal vaginal bleeding
Pelvic pain

17. Oral cancer

Oral cancer is any type of cancer that develops in the oral cavity: palate, tongue, lips, gums... The risk factors associated with this type of cancer are: smoking (including chewing tobacco) , alcoholism, weakened immune system, excessive sun exposure to the lips, and infection with the human papillomavirus (HPV).

The most common symptoms that indicate that the patient has this type of cancer are:

Mouth pain
No wound healing
Bumps in the oral cavity
Loss of dental support
Difficulty swallowing
ear pain
Patches of pus inside the mouth

18. Central nervous system cancer

Cancer in the central nervous system usually occurs in

the brain, where a group of cells in the brain begins to grow abnormally.

There are a wide variety of brain tumors, and although the causes are not very clear, there are certain risk factors, in particular exposure to ionizing radiation (such as that used in radiotherapy) and the presence of a family history .

Symptoms of central nervous system cancer depend a lot on the characteristics of the tumor, its location, and its size; Although, as a rule, they are as follows:

Increasingly intense and frequent headaches
Nausea and vomiting
Loss of mobility in extremities
Vision and hearing loss
Problems with maintaining balance
Speech difficulties
Personality changes
Seizures

19. Ovarian cancer

This type of cancer develops in the ovaries, although the fact that it is usually detected when it has already spread to the abdomen or pelvis makes treatment more complicated.

Although the causes are not known with certainty, the risk factors are: advanced age (usually occurs after 50 years), family history and genetic disorders, hormonal treatments (usually due to lack of estrogen) and the number of periods during a woman's fertile life.

The most common symptoms of ovarian cancer are:

Weightloss
Polyuria (need to urinate frequently)
Pelvic pain
abdominal swelling
Constipation
Quick feeling of satiety

20. Gallbladder cancer

This type of cancer develops in the gallbladder, an organ that stores bile, a liquid product produced by the liver with the function of helping to digest food.

Although the exact causes are not known, there are associated risk factors: female gender, advanced age, suffering from other gallbladder diseases and having suffered from gallstones in the past.

The most common symptoms associated with gallbladder cancer are:

Jaundice (yellowing of the skin)
Abdominal pain and swelling
Fever
Weightloss
Nausea

II.   The importance of early detection

If you regularly experience any of these symptoms or if you are not sure if you have developed one of these cancers, make an appointment with your doctor as

soon as possible.
Early detection greatly increases the chances of successful treatment.

Chapter 5: Cancer screening and detection

Early diagnosis of a malignant tumor is essential to treat it in time and cure the patient. These are the most common tests in the detection of cancer.

Our body is made up of a set of cells invisible to the naked eye. They are grouped together forming tissues, and these, in turn, give rise to organs which are the building blocks of complex systems with which we can breathe, think or digest the food we eat.

These cells must divide to replace those that are already old or dead, and thus maintain the optimal functioning of the organism in balance. Sometimes the control mechanisms fail and that's where we talk about cancer.

If cells begin to divide uncontrollably, they can lead to tumors. In case they have the ability to invade (i.e. produce metastases) and destroy other tissues, these tumors will be malignant.

The problem with cancer is that there are several types, depending on the area affected and the molecular factors involved in its development.

A recurring question of many patients is, undoubtedly, how the appearance of malignant tumors can be detected.

And there is no doubt, as the Spanish Association against Cancer explains, that this disease is treated as "one more" at the time of diagnosis. Medical professionals must first assess the patient's medical history, in order to study the family or personal history, as well as to know their lifestyle habits.

After this first analysis, and from the first suspicions

of a malignant tumour, the detection of cancer is mainly based on three types of tests: analytical (blood, urine, etc.), imaging and direct evaluation of the affected tissues.

I. Biomarkers : molecular clues to detect cancer

In the first case, blood tests can be clear signs that something is wrong with our body. The study of various biomarkers (such as protein CA-125 in ovarian cancer, PSA in prostate cancer or ACE in colon cancer) can be good clues to diagnose the disease and , in some cases, help plan treatment.

These markers are substances present in tissues or fluids such as blood or urine, which are produced by benign cells, although in much lower quantities than in the case of cancerous cells.

Its analysis is fundamental, and in fact there are more and more centers and companies specializing in molecular diagnostics.

Photographing the tumor may be key
biomarker studies using blood or urine tests, we have "indirect" indices, which do not always offer good results. Sometimes benign cells can abnormally produce certain molecular markers, without this indicating that we have developed a tumor.

Other times, in the early stages of cancer development, it is not so easy to determine the abnormalities in the aforementioned tests.

What to do then? Medicine, fortunately, has developed imaging studies that can be very useful in identifying the tumor mass. Using x-ray radiography, for example, we see bones as white areas and organs with air (like the lungs) as large dark pockets.

Mammography is also a type of X-ray, essential in this case in the detection and diagnosis of breast cancer.

Other imaging tests, such as magnetic resonance imaging or computed tomography (scan) can be performed by delivering contrast, because tumor cells absorb more of this substance than the patient's healthy cells.

In the case of scintigraphy, radioisotopes (iodine or technetium) are used, and this allows us to see very small lesions. There are other ways to "photograph" the possible existence of tumors, such as ultrasound, endoscopy and other types of tomography.

Making invisible tumor cells visible

As we explained at the beginning, our cells (healthy and tumor) are invisible to the naked eye, so to check how they are we need the help of a microscope.

The microscopic analysis of the tissue, extracted from the patient by biopsy (or cytology in the case of gynecological examinations), will be the one that will confirm or invalidate the malignancy.

The specimens that the pathologist must examine are sometimes subjected to other tests (beyond microscopic analysis of the cells). Methods such as immunohistochemistry, fluorescence in situ hybridization or RT-PCR seek to dive inside the "suspect" cells themselves, evaluating the chromosomes or genetic sequences themselves to confirm or refute the diagnosis.

There is no doubt that over the past few years research has made significant advances in the detection of cancer. An early diagnosis of this disease is essential to combat it and thus ensure the survival and total recovery of affected patients.

II.   Cancer detection

1. What is a detection?

A screening is a medical evaluation that is carried out outside of a known pathological situation. These tests can help detect disease at an early stage, before symptoms appear.

2. What is the name of the cancer screening test?

The test to detect cancer is known as cancer detection. These tests may include blood tests, X-rays, ultrasounds, biopsies, and other medical procedures.

3. Why is early detection of cancer important?

Early detection of cancer can significantly improve a person's survival and quality of life. Early detection tests can detect cancer before symptoms appear. This allows treatments to be more effective and less aggressive.

4. What types of cancer can be detected?

Some of the more common cancers that can be detected early include:

Lung cancer: This test looks for human papillomavirus (HPV) DNA in the mucus cells of the cervix.

Breast cancer: This test involves a physical examination of the breast, as well as a breast X-ray and a diagnostic test to detect the tumor.

Colorectal cancer: This test uses blood tests to detect cancerous proteins in the intestine.

Cervical Cancer: This test includes cytology cell analysis to detect abnormal changes in the cells of the cervix.

Prostate cancer: This test includes a blood test to detect the consequences of prostate cancer in the blood.

5. Where can I get a cancer screening test?

If you want to get tested for cancer, you should talk

to your doctor to see if it's right for you. Your doctor can recommend the best cancer screening test for you, based on your age, gender, and medical history.

6. Common exam types

Here are some of the most common tests:

Breast cancer screening: A breast cancer screening exam includes magnifying glass, MRI and blood test to detect the presence of cancerous antigens. This test is appropriate for women over 40.

Screening for cervical cancer: A screening for cervical cancer includes a flow test to detect the presence of abnormal cells and a flow test to detect the presence of human papillomavirus (HPV). This test is recommended for women over the age of 18.

Gastric cancer screening: A gastric cancer screening includes a blood test to check for albumin, a genetic test to check for genetic changes, and a CT scan to check for tumors. This test is recommended for people of any age who have a family history of gastric cancer.

Screening for prostate cancer: A screening test for prostate cancer includes a prostate-specific antigen (PSA) test to detect the presence of cancerous antigens in the blood and a digital rectal examination to detect the presence of tumors. This test is appropriate for men over 50.

7. Who should take this test?

Cancer screening is especially important for people who are at higher risk of developing cancer, such as older adults, those with a family history of cancer, and those whose genetic changes increase their risk of cancer.

8. Category of cancer screening test ?

Cancer screening is a medical procedure used to diagnose certain disorders in the body. These tests vary depending on the affected organ. It can detect intracellular changes that are not visible to the naked eye. Cancer screening falls into the following general categories:

- Imaging studies
- Genetic tests
- Biopsy
- Tumor markers

There are several types of tests that can be used to detect cancer, depending on the type of cancer. These may include:

General physical examinations. Healthcare professionals can use general physical exams to look for any signs of cancer in the neck, abdomen, and other common sites where tumors are.

CT scan. CT scans create detailed images of the inside of the body. This technique can be used to detect tumors.

Blood tests for tumor markers. Tumor markers are substances produced by tumors and released into the bloodstream. Patients may have blood tests to check their levels of these substances.

III.　Cancer symptoms that many ignore

Prevention and early detection are fundamental in the fight against cancer. Therefore, before any symptom that seems abnormal or generates concern, we must consult a specialist to evaluate it.

Knowing the possible symptoms of cancer that may occur is essential for going to the doctor for a checkup.

It should be noted that we should not be afraid because some of those we are going to mention occur, sporadically, but when they occur frequently with other discomforts, and prevent normal life.

Concerns:
Unusual tissue nodules, blisters and swelling.

It should be remembered that cancerous tumors are often painless, especially in the early stages of the disease. Particular attention should be paid to the neck, the testicles in men and the mammary glands in women, as well as the armpits.

-Prolonged cough, shortness of breath or difficulty swallowing.

-Changes in bowel habits.

-Sudden onset of constipation or, on the contrary,

frequent episodes of diarrhea, especially if traces of blood are visible in the stool.

-Unexpected bleeding – including light bleeding from the vagina, rectum, blood in the urine or sputum when coughing.

- **Unexplained weight loss** . If you have unexpectedly noticeably lost weight in a relatively short period of time (about two months), this is cause for concern and a trip to the doctor. In addition to cancer, sudden weight loss can signal a serious thyroid problem or diabetes.

- **Chronic fatigue and catastrophic lack of energy** for usual things, despite healthy and normal sleep. Usually, if the cause of chronic fatigue is the onset of cancer, the patient also has other symptoms.

- **Unexplained pain:** of any nature and frequency: acute attacks and pain; both chronic and appearing only occasionally.

The appearance of new moles or the transformation of existing moles: changes in size, shape or color; hardening of the surface of the birthmark or any discharge.

Problems with urination , including more frequent or more urgent urges and difficulty or pain in the process.

Unusual breast changes. A cause for concern may be an unexpected change in the size or shape of the mammary glands, as well as changes in sensations to touch, including on the skin of the breasts, or pain.

Loss of appetite. If your hunger has gone down for a long time and you've started eating less than usual, that's also a warning sign, even if you don't have any other symptoms.

Non-healing sore or other sore, especially in the mouth.

Chronic heartburn or other regular digestive disorders: nausea, vomiting, bloating and others.

Profuse sweating at night.

IV.   Symptoms

One of the main ways to fight cancer is to catch it early. Sometimes, because we are very busy, we forget to have our annual medical examinations and wait weeks before going to the consultation if we are in pain.

Cancer has early symptoms that many of us are unaware of. Therefore, it is important to know them to take them into account.

1. Possible symptoms of cancer (in men and women)

Although talking about cancer can cause some fear, it is essential to be well informed about the subject so that, in the event of a change in the state of health, we go to the doctor and discuss our concerns.

a) Weightloss

Another possible symptom of cancer is sudden weight loss, for no apparent reason and without making any changes in diet or exercise habits, may be associated with a certain type of cancer.

b) Frequent cough

Frequent coughing cannot just be caused by an allergy or a change in temperature. It can also be caused by more serious illnesses, such as cancer.

If you constantly have a cold, even if you don't smoke, you should see a doctor. Cancer of the lung, throat or larynx can be prepared. You should also watch out for chest pain and symptoms similar to severe bronchitis (discomfort spreads to the shoulders or under the arms).

c) Frequent fever

Leukemia is a type of cancer that grows in the bone marrow and attacks blood cells. Diseased or abnormal white blood cells are produced, which affects the body's ability to prevent or fight infection.

d) Joint pain

It is true that joints can become inflamed and painful due to sudden movement, overexertion or poor posture, but it can also be a sign of something more serious like bone cancer. If joint pain does not go away, it may be time to see a doctor.

e) Bruises that won't heal, another possible symptom of cancer

If we hit something or fall, it is normal to have bruises or bruises. The problem lies in their appearance for no apparent reason or in a very slow healing process (when they change color until they disappear).

It can be a sign of unhealthy platelets and red blood cells and even leukemia which does not allow blood to carry oxygen or clot properly.

f) Various skin changes

According to experts from the American Cancer Association, there are skin changes that can be a sign of several types of cancer (not just the skin):

Itch. Excessive hair growth.
Darkening (hyperpigmentation).
Yellowing of the skin and eyes (jaundice).
Changes in the male reproductive system
If you notice a lump, inflammation or pain (among other changes) in the testicles, it is necessary to go to the doctor to determine the reason. Testicular cancer is one of the fastest growing. According to doctors, men between the ages of 15 and 55 can do a self-examination at home to monitor changes.

Also, do not underestimate problems with urination: need to go to the bathroom all the time, difficulty in starting to urinate or little urine. It can be a symptom of prostate cancer, a disease that occurs mostly in men over 50.

2. Possible symptoms of cancer in women

Now let's look at the possible symptoms of cancer in women. It should be noted that they are not the only ones that should be taken into account when taking concerns to the doctor.

a) Bloating

10% of the population suffer from regular bloating, especially women. This common condition is linked to premenstrual syndrome, indigestion, or gas buildup.

But if the inflammation persists for more than two weeks (and pregnancy is ruled out) and is associated with weight loss or bleeding, it could be one of the symptoms of cancer. Therefore, it is advisable to consult a doctor to find out if it is ovarian cancer.

b) Bleeding between periods

During the menstrual cycle, the woman may experience bleeding even when she does not have her period. However, when it happens very often and several times in the same month, it can be due to a hormonal problem, stress, inflammation of the cervix or endometrial cancer.

c) Breast changes

As with men, women can also have their breasts examined while bathing or in front of the mirror. The appearance of bumps (which may extend to the armpits), suppuration of the nipple, skin changes or pain outside the menstrual period should be analyzed.

Chapter 6: Cancer treatment

One in six deaths worldwide is due to cancer. It is the second leading cause of death worldwide, behind cardiovascular disease.

8.8 million people died from this disease in 2015. Since statistics indicate that approximately 1 in 3 women and 1 in 2 men will develop some type of cancer during their lifetime, cancer research is a primary public health problem.

The fight against cancer
Thanks to this work of researchers, treatments have been developed and continue to be developed, which have made it possible to increase survival by 20% over the past twenty years.
This improvement in the expectations of people affected by cancer stems from increasingly specific and effective treatments.

Cancer research is the driving force behind the reduction of mortality caused by cancer, carrying out increasingly effective prevention and transforming it into a curable or, at least, chronic disease.

We will examine the treatments currently available, analyzing their characteristics and their differences.

I.   What are the types of treatments to

fight cancer?

Thanks to the synergy of various specialties in biology and medicine, we have succeeded in developing many types of treatments to fight against these malignant tumors.

The treatment a patient receives depends on several factors, especially the type of cancer you have developed and how advanced it is.

The prescription of one treatment or another is determined by the stage of diagnosis. This is why precise detection of cancer is essential in order to then apply a specific treatment depending on the nature of the tumor and the stage in which it is.

The importance of this diagnosis lies in the fact that each type of cancer requires a specific protocol which can also include the use of several therapies at the same time, combining treatments. In fact, some of the most common cancers, such as breast and colon cancer, have high cure rates if diagnosed early and accurately.

As in any area of the clinic, these treatments have the main objective of curing the cancer or, failing that, prolonging the patient's life as much as possible.

In addition to this obvious goal, these therapies should also focus on improving the patient's quality of life, which can be achieved by offering palliative care, relieving the symptoms of the disease, as well as psychological support . and social.

These are the types of treatment currently used to

fight malignant tumors.

1. Surgery

Surgery is the therapy in which a surgeon removes the tumor from the body of a cancer patient. Many people affected by a malignant tumor are treated with this technique, which is advisable to practice when dealing with solid tumors contained in a limited area of the body.

This is why it cannot be used for leukemia (blood cancer) or tumors that have metastasized, ie spread to other areas of the body.

It's a local treatment, so targeting other areas of the body that don't have cancer is risk-free. Although surgery is sometimes the only treatment a patient will receive, this technique must often be used in conjunction with other treatments.

The risks of this technique are mainly pain and the possibility of infection. The degree of pain the patient will experience will depend on the extent of the operation and the area the surgeons worked on.

In case of infections, the risk of suffering from them will be reduced if you follow the advice of cleaning and disinfecting the wound.

2. Radiotherapy

Radiation therapy uses radioactive X-rays, particles or seeds to kill cancer cells. Cells of this type grow and divide faster than normal cells in the body.

Because radiation is more harmful to rapidly growing cells, radiation therapy damages cancer cells more than normal cells. This prevents cancer cells from growing and dividing, which leads to cell death.

The two main types of radiotherapy are:
External radiotherapy. This is the most common method. In it, X-rays or particles are directed at the tumor from outside the body.

Internal radiotherapy . This form delivers radiation inside your body. It can be applied through radioactive seeds that are placed in or near the tumor; a liquid or pill you swallow; or through a vein (intravenously or IV).

3. Chemotherapy

Chemotherapy includes all treatments to fight cancer that base their action on the use of drugs that stop or slow down the growth of cancer cells.

This therapy is used to treat many types of cancer and may be the only treatment they receive. However, its widespread use is due to the fact that chemotherapy is usually the step before the application of other treatments.
It is often used to shrink the tumor before surgery or radiation therapy, in addition to other treatments, or even to kill cancer cells that may remain after surgery.

Like radiotherapy, the action of chemotherapy is not specific to cancer cells, thus affecting the growth of healthy cells that divide rapidly, such as those that line the intestines or those that grow hair.
This is why the most common side effects of this

therapy are fatigue, hair loss, nausea, mouth ulcers and vomiting. But nevertheless, these side effects often get better or go away after treatment is finished.

4. Immunotherapy

Immunotherapy is the treatment of helping the immune system fight cancer. It is considered a biological therapy in which substances produced by organisms are used to treat tumors.

Although this therapy has been approved to treat many types of cancer, it is still not used as much as surgery, chemotherapy or radiation therapy.
Future projections indicate that as more clinical trials are conducted, its use will become much more widespread.

One of the reasons why cancer cells grow and are not killed by our body is that they have the ability to hide from the immune system.
The action of immunotherapy is to mark these cancerous cells and then alert the immune system to where they are so that, also reinforced by treatment, it can naturally fight the tumour.

This therapy is usually given intravenously, so the side effects are related to our reaction to this injection: pain, redness and flu-like symptoms (fever, chills, weakness, nausea, vomiting, etc.).

5. Targeted treatment

Targeted therapy is a type of treatment that acts on

the functioning of cancer cells, which affects properties related to its growth, division and spread.

It is in this therapy that the need to continue to study the nature of malignant tumors is most reflected , because by knowing them thoroughly, we can find new targets to block the harmful characteristics of these cells.

This treatment consists of the use of micromolecular drugs, which penetrate into cancer cells and inhibit their functions, or monoclonal antibodies, which adhere to the surface of cancer cells to also inhibit their properties.

It is indicated for patients with a certain type of cancer with cells that we know well and for which there is a target on which these drugs can act. To determine this, it will be necessary to perform a biopsy, that is, to remove part of the tumor and analyze it.

Biopsy carries risks, which, together with the fact that cancer cells can become resistant to drugs and there are negative side effects, is why this therapy is not fully widespread.

6. Hormone therapy

Hormonal or endocrine therapy is a treatment used to fight breast and prostate cancer because the cancer cells that cause them use hormones (that our own body generates) to grow.

This therapy can block the body's ability to produce

hormones or interfere with the way hormones behave in the body.

Both actions aim to prevent cancer cells from having their own growth substrate and thus stop their expansion or, at least, relieve the patient's symptoms.

The side effects of this treatment are given by the hormonal inhibition suffered by the patient: hot flushes, fatigue, breast pain, alterations in the female cycle, vaginal dryness, nausea, loss of sexual appetite, weak bones, etc. .

7. Stem cell transplants

Stem cell transplantation is a type of treatment that does not work directly against cancer, but rather helps the patient regain the ability to generate stem cells after chemotherapy or radiation therapy.

In chemotherapy or radiotherapy at very high doses, blood cells are destroyed. With this transplant, stem cells are transfused into the bloodstream, traveling to the bone marrow and then replacing cells that died during treatment.

The patient thus regains the ability to produce white blood cells, red blood cells and platelets, essential components of the circulatory system.

Although its possible use in other types of cancer is being studied, this treatment is currently used to help patients with leukemia and lymphoma, although it is also often used in patients with neuroblastomas and multiple myeloma.

The negative effects of this treatment are bleeding, increased risk of infection and possible rejection of donated tissues, so it is necessary to ensure that the cells received are as compatible as possible with the patient.

8. Hyperthermia

Hyperthermia uses heat to damage and kill cancer cells without harming normal cells.

It can be used for:

A small area of cells, like a tumor
Body parts, such as an organ or limb
The whole body
The heat is given by a machine outside the body or by a needle or tube placed in the tumour.

9. Laser therapy

Laser therapy uses a very narrow, focused beam of light to destroy cancer cells. Laser therapy can be used for:

Destroy tumors and precancerous neoplasms
Shrinking tumors that block the stomach, colon, or esophagus
Help treat symptoms of cancer, such as bleeding
Seal nerve endings after surgery to reduce pain
Seal the lymph vessels after surgery to reduce swelling and prevent tumor cells from spreading

Laser therapy is often delivered through a thin, lighted tube that is placed inside the body. The thin fibers at the end of the tube direct the light to the cancer cells. Lasers are also used on the skin.

In most cases, lasers are used along with other types of cancer treatments such as radiation therapy and chemotherapy.

10. Photodynamic therapy

photodynamic therapy , a person is injected with a drug that is sensitive to a particular type of light. The drug stays in cancer cells longer than it stays in healthy cells.
A doctor then directs light from a laser or other source at the cancer cells. The light turns the drug into a substance that kills cancer cells.

11. The importance of precision medicine

Traditionally, the selection of therapies to treat cancer has been similar to a mathematical equation: depending on the type of cancer and its stage, the treatment is chosen.

Despite the obvious successes of this approach, the relatively recent discovery that tumors undergo genetic changes as they grow and spread, and that these are different for each patient, has led researchers to focus research on the direction of so-called precision medicine.

This precision medicine stems from the need to select the treatments most likely to help the patient based on the genetic variables of cancer cells.

Targeted therapy is a type of cancer treatment that uses drugs or other substances to identify and precisely target certain types of cancer cells.
Targeted therapy may be used alone or in combination with other treatments, such as traditional or standard chemotherapy, surgery, or radiation therapy .
If targeted therapy is part of your treatment plan, knowing how it works and what to expect can help you prepare for treatment and make informed decisions about your healthcare.

Conclusion

Cancer is a complex disease that can affect anyone at any time of life. It is a disease that can be caused by many different factors, including environment, heredity, and lifestyle.

Fortunately, thanks to medical and scientific advances, there are many effective treatment options available today to fight cancer.

In this practical guide to the symptoms, causes and treatments of cancerous diseases, we have explored the different facets of this devastating disease.

We looked at the main types of cancers, the symptoms that go with them and the associated risk factors. We also looked at the different treatments available, including chemotherapy, radiotherapy and surgery.

One of the main messages of this book is that prevention is the best weapon against cancer. By adopting a healthy lifestyle, avoiding risky behaviors such as smoking and excessive alcohol consumption, and having regular checkups, people can significantly reduce their risk of developing cancer.

However, even with proper prevention, it is still possible to develop cancer. In these cases, it is important to see a doctor as soon as possible for proper diagnosis and treatment . Treatment options can be very different depending on the type of cancer and the severity of the disease.

In some cases, simple surgery may be enough to remove the tumor, while in others, a combination of chemotherapy, radiation therapy and targeted therapies may be needed.

It is also important to emphasize that the fight against cancer is a process that requires emotional and psychological support. People with cancer, as well as their families and friends, can benefit from the help of mental health professionals to deal with the emotional and psychological challenges associated with the disease.

Over the years, many people have been affected by cancer, either directly or indirectly. Celebrities such as Patrick Swayze , Steve Jobs and John McCain have all succumbed to the disease, and millions of others have been affected as well.

However, thanks to the efforts of researchers, doctors and patients, significant progress has been made in the fight against cancer.

Examples of these advances include the introduction of new targeted therapies, which can attack cancer cells while leaving healthy cells intact.

Immunotherapies are also revolutionizing the fight against cancer by using the body's immune system to attack cancer cells. Additionally, advances in technology have allowed for more accurate diagnoses and more effective treatments, as well as less invasive procedures.

However, there is still a long way to go to defeat cancer. Researchers work tirelessly to discover new treatments, improve existing treatments and find ways to prevent cancer.

Awareness campaigns and screening programs are also essential to enable people to take preventive measures and detect the disease at an early stage.

Another important aspect of the fight against cancer is access to health care. Unfortunately, many people around the world do not have access to the treatments they need due to financial, geographical or social constraints.

It is essential that governments, health organizations and patient advocacy groups work together to ensure that all cancer patients have access to the care they need, regardless of where they live, their status socio-economic or ethnic origin.

Finally, it is important to recognize that the fight against cancer is a collective effort. Patients, healthcare professionals, researchers, healthcare organizations and communities must all work together to prevent, detect and treat disease.

Patients should be encouraged to take an active role in their own treatment by asking questions, seeking information, and seeking emotional support. Healthcare professionals must be equipped with the latest knowledge and best practices to provide top quality care.

Healthcare organizations should support research and awareness and provide resources to help patients and their families.

In conclusion, cancer is a complex and devastating disease that can affect anyone. However, thanks to scientific and medical advances, there are now many effective treatment options available to combat the disease.

Prevention is the best weapon against cancer, but it is also essential to consult a doctor as soon as possible in the event of symptoms.

The fight against cancer is a process that requires emotional and psychological support, as well as quality health care.

By working together, we can make great strides in the fight against cancer and improve the lives of patients and their families around the world.

Contents

Fighting cancer: a practical guide to the symptoms, causes and treatments of cancerous diseases